Contents

The changing face of renal medicine in the UK

future of the specialty

Report of a Working Party 2007

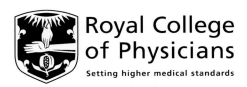

Royal College of Physicians
Setting higher medical standards

The Renal Association

The Royal College of Physicians of London

The Royal College of Physicians plays a leading role in the delivery of high quality patient care by setting standards of medical practice and promoting clinical excellence. We provide physicians in the UK and overseas with education, training and support throughout their careers. As an independent body representing over 20,000 Fellows and Members worldwide, we advise and work with government, the public, patients and other professions to improve health and healthcare.

The Renal Association

The Renal Association is the professional association of renal physicians and renal scientists in the UK. It seeks to improve the health of people with kidney disease by developing guidelines for clinical care, and by disseminating the information gathered by its UK Renal Registry, as well as by promoting research into renal disease and providing specialist professional education.

Citation of this document: Royal College of Physicians. *The changing face of renal medicine in the UK: the future of the specialty.* Report of a Working Party. London: RCP, 2007.

ROYAL COLLEGE OF PHYSICIANS OF LONDON
11 St Andrews Place, London NW1 4LE
www.rcplondon.ac.uk
Registered Charity No 210508

THE RENAL ASSOCIATION
Durford Mill, Petersfield, Hampshire GU31 5AZ
www.renal.org

ISBN 978-1-86016-296-1

Review date: 2015

Typeset by Dan-Set Graphics, Telford, Shropshire

Printed in Great Britain by Sarum ColourView Group, Salisbury, Wiltshire

Preface

This Working Party is reporting at a time of exciting change in renal medicine. The publication of National Service Frameworks for Renal Services in England and Wales offers a unique opportunity to develop the provision of high-quality patient-centred renal services. There are pivotal changes promoting the chance to develop collaborative services with primary care, palliative care and other specialist teams. Multiprofessional team working, in which renal medicine has always led the way, continues to expand and challenges long-established medical roles.

Against this backdrop the career goals and expectations of young doctors are changing and the traditional model of a full-time consultant working in a 'long hours culture' has become less attractive.

Members of the Working Party believe that renal medicine continues to offer a varied and satisfying career, combining the clinical challenge of complex illness with the holistic care of chronic disease, as well as the intellectual challenge which continues to put the specialty at the forefront of academic medicine.

This report makes recommendations which we regard as crucial to taking the opportunities for the continuing development of renal medicine in the UK. We believe our report will assist the following groups:

- ► commissioners of renal services

- ► NHS trusts that are providers of renal services

- ► locality renal networks

- ► the Specialty Advisory Committee (SAC) for Renal Medicine and others concerned with the training of renal physicians

- ► Department of Health Renal Advisory Group and other bodies charged with overseeing implementation of the National Service Framework for Renal Services in England, and equivalent framework advice in other parts of the UK

- ► kidney patient associations.

I acknowledge gratefully the energetic and thoughtful contributions of all members of the Working Party, especially the wise perspectives of Bob Price, a member of the Royal College of Physician's Patient and Carer Network, and Dr Paul Rylance who drafted this document. Kim BIllingham gave faultless administrative support to the Working Party on behalf of the Royal College of Physicians.

November 2006
John Monson
Chair, Working Party

Members of the Working Party

John Monson *(Chair)*
Emeritus Professor of Clinical Endocrinology and Consultant Physician, St Bartholomew's and the Royal London Hospitals

Lindsey Barker
Consultant Nephrologist, Royal Berkshire Hospital

Gordon Bell
Consultant Nephrologist and Clinical Director of Renal Medicine, Royal Liverpool University Hospital

John Feehally
Consultant Nephrologist, University Hospitals of Leicester; Honorary Professor of Renal Medicine, University of Leicester; President, Renal Association

Tim Goodship
Professor of Renal Medicine, University of Newcastle upon Tyne

Bob Price
Patient and Carer Network Representative Royal College of Physicians

Paul Rylance
Consultant Nephrologist, Royal Wolverhampton Hospitals; Chair, Society for DGH Nephrologists

Executive summary and recommendations

Executive summary

Against a background of changes to both the medical workforce and the pattern of day-to-day clinical work for renal physicians, the Working Party makes recommendations on the delivery of patient care, medical staffing and the provision and commissioning of renal services. We have consulted all relevant stakeholders and when possible have used their input to make clear recommendations (see section 1.3). Furthermore, all stakeholders were extremely helpful in viewing the totality of the remit rather than restricting themselves to their own area of expertise.

Service provision

Recent growth in renal services has been predominantly in district general hospitals (DGHs). There should be little distinction made between the range of services (including supporting services) provided by renal units in DGHs and those in traditional teaching hospitals, other than acute transplantation. We propose two models for renal units: a renal and transplant unit (RTU) providing a visiting service for smaller hospitals and a renal unit (RU), which might also support smaller neighbouring hospitals. In many localities an RTU will work within a renal network which also contains one or more RUs.

Medical staffing

As the service need grows, we recommend that there should be a substantial increase in consultant numbers, particularly in RUs. A renal unit may be established with two consultants, but should have a minimum of four to become autonomous. Commitment to general internal medicine (GIM) should not be expected throughout a consultant career. Staff grades and associate specialists should be actively encouraged to join the Specialist Register, either by re-entering specialty training or via Article 14 of the regulations of the Postgraduate Medical Education and Training Board (PMETB). Establishing dialysis medicine as an approved specialty to which PMETB can offer specialist registration may be of particular interest to this group. To promote renal medicine as a career, the perception of an intensive 'long hours' specialty should be offset by offering a positive experience to both medical students and foundation year trainees. Specialty training should be streamlined across the involved organisations, particularly to ensure seamless educational approval and local funding. As working patterns reduce exposure to experiential learning, this will need to be complemented by competency-based training with sufficient resources in postgraduate medical education and web-based learning. We recommend that there should be opportunities after completion of training in renal medicine to develop accredited subspecialty expertise in dialysis medicine, critical care nephrology, interventional nephrology, and transplant medicine. We encourage secondment to obtain high-quality research experience and recommend the establishment of a UK clinical research network for renal disease. Through-out the medical workforce, flexible training opportunities should be expanded, fully funded and part of the mainstream service provision.

Patient-centred care

In the provision of patient-centred care, we support the continuing expansion of extended competency-based roles for all health professionals in the renal multiprofessional team, and redefinition of the roles of doctors within that team. The increasing emphasis on early detection of chronic kidney disease (CKD) and the provision of non-dialysis care for some patients with advanced renal failure will require specific links with primary and relevant specialist secondary care services. Support services for renal units must include specialist expertise in diagnostic and interventional radiology, and pathology expertise sufficient to provide an urgent diagnostic service and routine clinico-pathological meetings. All renal units require an up-to-date clinical information system with appropriate informatics support. It will be essential that NHS Connecting for Health provides at the very least continuation of current functionality for renal units and for the UK Renal Registry. The transfer of young people with renal disease to adult services is a time of high risk and the need for a streamlined process is paramount.

Commissioning

There is geographical inequality in the provision of UK renal services. We recommend that specialised commissioning of renal services becomes more effective, using locality networks, needs assessment and prioritised investment. Tariffs for renal service will be complex, must be developed with full clinical engagement, and should include costing for pre-dialysis care and non-dialysis care of patients with advanced renal failure.

RECOMMENDATIONS

Provision of renal services in the UK

R1   **We recommend** two preferred models for renal units: either a renal and transplant unit (RTU) providing a visiting service for surrounding DGHs, or a renal unit (RU) which might also provide a visiting service to smaller neighbouring DGHs. A population of 0.5 million is typically sufficient to justify the need for an RU, although local geographical factors might influence the size of population served.

R2   **We recommend** that there should be little distinction made between RUs (usually in DGHs) and RTUs in the traditional teaching hospitals, in the range of services provided, other than acute transplantation. In addition, there should be no distinction in the need for supporting services (for example surgery, imaging, and laboratory services) nor in the staffing requirements in the renal unit of both career grades and training grades of medical staff and other health professionals.

Medical staffing of renal units

Consultants

R3   **We recommend** that there should be a substantial increase in the number of consultant renal physicians in the UK, particularly in RUs with a GIM commitment. This should include positive support for consultants wishing to work flexibly. We recommend that one consultant renal physician (who has additional responsibilities for general medicine) is required per 75 renal replacement therapy patients or one full-time consultant renal physician for 100 renal replacement therapy patients. If a consultant is responsible for the care of patients with established renal transplants, a higher number of patients per consultant is appropriate. These figures could underestimate the requirement in RUs where consultants have a major commitment to GIM and where there are usually fewer specialty registrars.

R4   **We recommend** that a minimum of two consultant appointments is necessary to establish a new renal unit, and a minimum of four consultants is required before a renal unit can be autonomous and provide all services other than acute transplantation. Autonomy should usually be attained within five years and during the interim period the unit should be supported by a managed clinical network.

R5   **We recommend** that a commitment to GIM should not be expected to continue throughout a consultant career. The career development of individuals may result in their taking over other responsibilities such as management and teaching, and in changes in their clinical commitments including GIM.

Staff grades and associate specialists

R6   **We recommend** that staff grades and associates specialists should be actively encouraged to join the Specialist Register, if necessary re-entering specialty training to do so. Flexible training should be available to facilitate such career development.

R7   **We recommend** that there is clarification of entry to the Specialist Register via Article 14 of the PMETB for doctors trained solely in the UK, who might currently be excluded from the Specialist Register under these regulations.

R8   **We recommend** that dialysis medicine becomes an approved specialty to which PMETB can offer specialist registration

Recruitment and training

R9   **We recommend** that interest in renal medicine as a career is encouraged early in training by ensuring that medical students have a positive experience of the specialty during their undergraduate training, and then by offering experience in renal medicine during the foundation years.

R10   **We recommend** that the process of organisation and monitoring of specialty training is streamlined, with clearer description of the responsibilities of the involved organisations.

R11   **We recommend** that local funding issues should not delay the establishment of specialty training posts which have received workforce and educational approval.

R12   **We recommend** that opportunities for flexible training for doctors in training are expanded, are part of mainstream service provision and are readily funded.

R13   **We recommend** that competency-based training is developed to complement (but not replace) experiential learning, with sufficient resources for postgraduate medical education including the increased availability of web-based distance learning, to ensure that support for competency-based training does not compromise patient care.

R14   **We recommend** that opportunities be developed to share modules of training with other specialties, for example diabetes and cardiology.

R15   **We recommend** that there should be opportunities after completion of renal medicine training for additional experience enabling renal physicians to develop accredited subspecialty expertise in dialysis medicine, critical care nephrology, interventional nephrology, and transplant medicine.

Academic renal medicine

R16   **We recommend** that trainees are given the opportunity to undertake original research with the aim of achieving a higher degree during specialty training. We recognise that full-time research will not be undertaken by all trainees, but all should have exposure to research methodology. We recommend that trainees also avail themselves of opportunities to develop experience in other aspects of professional work, including education and management.

R17   **We recommend** that there should be opportunities to undertake such training on a flexible basis.

R18   **We recommend** that a split of 50% academic:50% clinical is an appropriate balance in workload for academic nephrologists.

R19   **We recommend** the establishment of a UK clinical research network in renal disease.

Provision of patient-centred care

R20   **We recommend** that renal services are developed in line with the standards and markers of good practice in the National Framework for Renal Services for England and equivalent framework documents in other parts of the UK; ensuring that patient-centred, holistic care is available for all renal patients.

R21   **We recommend** the continuing expansion of competency-based training for all health professionals in the renal multiprofessional team, allowing extended roles for nurses and other practitioners.

R22   **We recommend** redefining the roles of doctors within the renal multiprofessional team wherever this is appropriate to the holistic care of patients and the professional development of other members of the team. A goal of this redefinition is to allow the most effective use of the specific skills of physicians in evaluation, diagnosis, and overall responsibility for patient management.

R23   **We recommend** the development of a subspecialty of transplant medicine.

R24   **We recommend** that all renal units have access to specialist expertise in diagnostic and interventional radiology.

R25   **We recommend** that renal pathology expertise should be available to all renal units sufficient to provide an urgent diagnostic service and routine clinico-pathological meetings, if necessary by remote videoconferencing.

R26   **We recommend** that all renal units have an electronic clinical information system with appropriate informatics support, and that plans are developed with NHS Connecting for Health to ensure continuation of functionality currently available in renal unit clinical information systems, and to ensure availability of necessary data for the work of the UK Renal Registry.

R27   **We recommend** the development of subspecialty training in clinical care nephrology in conjunction with intensive care medicine.

R28   **We recommend** that the transfer of young people from paediatrics to adult care should be a seamless multidisciplinary process.

R29   **We recommend** joint working between the renal multiprofessional team, primary care and relevant specialist secondary care services promoting integrated care for patients with chronic kidney disease (CKD), diabetes, vascular disease, and for elderly patients and those patients who require conservative or palliative care. Consultant renal physicians should play a key leadership role in these service developments. These services should be in line with available clinical practice guidelines, and should be fully funded.

Commissioning of renal services

R30   **We recommend** an increased emphasis on the need for effective commissioning of renal services through locality networks, supported by a robust assessment of need and a prioritised investment plan.

R31   **We recommend** that prevailing inequalities of provision of renal services are addressed, ensuring that the impact of ethnicity and social deprivation are properly identified when calculating funding.

R32   **We recommend** that the tariff for renal services should be developed to properly reflect the cost of the complex activities of chronic disease management in renal care. This will require in depth clinical engagement.

R33   **We recommend** that reference costs for pre-dialysis care and non-dialysis care of advanced renal failure are developed.

R34   **We recommend** that all providers of renal services (including the NHS and the independent sector) should conform to RCP/Renal Association standards of care. Care must be integrated and seamless. It is crucial that maintenance of standards of care across public and private providers is rigorously audited.

Glossary

Acute renal failure: sudden loss of kidney function, commonly associated with severe medical or surgical illnesses, which might require critical care unit treatment. Sudden deterioration in the function of already severely damaged kidneys can also cause acute renal failure.

Anaemia: in impaired renal function, reduced function of the bone marrow due to lack of the hormone erythropoietin results in anaemia and can be corrected by erythropoietin injections.

APD: automated peritoneal dialysis

Arteriovenous fistula: an artery and a vein joined in the patient's arm to provide a dilated vessel for needle insertion for haemodialysis.

Automated peritoneal dialysis: peritoneal dialysis performed overnight at home using an automated machine.

CAPD: continuous ambulatory peritoneal dialysis

Chronic kidney disease (CKD): evidence of chronic kidney damage with:

- ▶ normal renal function   stage 1, eGFR >90ml/min
- ▶ mild impairment   stage 2, eGFR 60–89ml/min
- ▶ moderate impairment   stage 3, eGFR 30–59ml/min
- ▶ severe impairment   stage 4, eGFR 15–29ml/min
- ▶ established renal failure or on dialysis   stage 5, eGFR <15ml/min.

Clinical network: a managed group of units collaborating to provide care for renal patients according to agreed national standards.

Combined kidney-pancreas transplant: simultaneous transplantation into a diabetic patient of a kidney and pancreas from the same deceased donor, so removing the need for both dialysis and insulin therapy.

Commissioning: the planning and purchase of clinical services by primary care trusts, strategic health authorities or hospital trusts.

Co-morbidity: presence of other medical conditions likely to effect either survival or quality of life of the patient.

Continuous ambulatory peritoneal dialysis: peritoneal dialysis performed using usually four exchanges of fluid per day.

Deceased donor: a kidney donated for transplantation by a patient, usually on a critical care unit, who has suffered irreversible brain death as determined by accepted brain death criteria.

DGH: district general hospital

Dialysis adequacy: the calculation of the amount of dialysis required, according to national or international standards, to adequately clear toxins accumulating as a result of renal failure.

Dialysis medicine: a subspecialty of renal medicine managing patients on haemodialysis and peritoneal dialysis and provided by doctors with additional specific training in these areas.

eGFR: estimated glomerular filtration rate: a calculation of glomerular filtration rate from the patient's serum creatinine, age, sex and ethnicity.

ESRD: end-stage renal disease

EWTD: European Work Time Directive

Foundation years: the training of junior doctors in the first two years following qualification.

General (internal) medicine (GIM): the provision of care for patients with a variety of medical conditions, particularly those with acute medical presentations.

Glomerular filtration rate (GFR): a more accurate estimation of renal function, best performed by a radio-isotopic technique, which is rarely used in clinical practice, but can be estimated by a calculation (see eGFR).

Graft: a plastic vessel surgically inserted as an alternative to an arteriovenous fistula; also called an arteriovenous (AV) graft. Graft can also refer to a kidney transplant.

Graft failure: the failure of a renal transplant, either because of acute rejection or chronic progressive damage to the transplant. May also refer to clotting of an arteriovenous graft.

Holistic care: the provision of all the needs of the patient, whether medical, psychological or social.

Hospital at Night: the provision of night-time care for hospital patients, in a number of specialties, by teams of doctors and other health professionals.

Interventional radiology: specialty where radiologists perform X-rays or scans in order to carry out renal biopsies, insert drainage tubes into kidneys or perform angioplasty (balloon dilatation) of renal arteries, as alternatives to surgical operations.

ISTC: Independent Sector Treatment Centre

JCHMT: Joint Committee for Higher Medical Training

Living donor: a kidney donated by a relative (living related) or a spouse, partner or friend (living unrelated) to a renal patient.

MMC: Modernising Medical Careers

Multi-organ failure: failure of the function of several organs, commonly including kidneys, associated with severe medical or surgical conditions.

NICE: National Institute for Health and Clinical Excellence

NSF: National Service Framework

NTN: national training numbers

Palliative care: care of a patient focussing on relieving symptoms rather than curing the underlying condition.

Patient pathway: a guideline or protocol for the multidisciplinary management and care of a medical condition.

Payment by Results: a national tariff system for hospital trusts, whereby trusts receive payment for the clinical activity and procedures they undertake.

PCT: primary care trust

PD: peritoneal dialysis

Percutaneous dialysis catheter: a double-lumen plastic catheter inserted in neck or upper leg vessels to allow haemodialysis in the absence of an arteriovenous fistula or a graft.

Peritoneal dialysis: a home dialysis technique where the patient drains dialysis fluid into the peritoneal cavity via a plastic peritoneal catheter.

PMETB: Postgraduate Medical Education and Training Board

pmp: per million population

QOF: Quality and Outcomes Framework

Renal bone disease: biochemical and hormonal abnormalities as a result of moderate to severe renal impairment, eventually causing alteration of the structure of bone.

Renal replacement therapy (RRT): the treatment of patients with established renal failure by haemodialysis, peritoneal dialysis or renal transplantation.

RTU: renal and transplant unit

RU: renal unit

SAC: Specialty Advisory Committee

Skill-mix: the collaborative and complementary skills of the multidisciplinary team.

SpR: specialist registrar, which will be replaced by the term specialty registrar (StR).

Transplant medicine: a subspecialty of renal medicine, involved in preparation of patients for renal transplantation, counselling potential living donors, and long-term follow-up of transplant patients after the transplant operation.

Transplantation: renal replacement therapy by a renal transplant, either from a living donor or a deceased donor.

Type 1 diabetes: diabetes mellitus, commonly but not exclusively with a younger age of onset, due to severe insulin deficiency.

Type 2 diabetes: diabetes mellitus, most commonly presenting in middle-aged and older adults, due to partial insulin deficiency and/or insulin resistance.

WTE: whole-time equivalent

1 Background and remit

The need for a Working Party

1.1   The size and distribution of the medical workforce in renal medicine in the UK is changing rapidly. Factors influencing these changes include:

▶ the increasing number of consultant appointments in renal medicine, an increasing proportion of whom work in district general hospitals (DGHs) with renal units (RUs), rather than in the larger traditional teaching hospitals with renal and transplant units (RTUs)

▶ the falling proportion of clinical academics in renal medicine, who previously made a substantial contribution to the clinical service and its development, and the difficulties in recruiting into academic medicine in the UK

▶ the decreasing contribution of renal physicians to general (internal) medicine (GIM)

▶ the increasing number of specialty registrars in renal medicine

▶ the increasing number of renal physicians who choose to work part time (the majority of whom are women) both during training and in career posts, as well as the recognition that the high-intensity work patterns typical of consultant renal physicians may not be appropriate for all consultants at all stages of their careers

▶ the key role played by staff grades and associate specialists in many renal units, and the impact for these doctors of the changing Postgraduate Medical Education and Training Board (PMETB) regulations about direct entry to the consultant grade

▶ the impact of both the European Working Time Directive (EWTD) on rotas, continuous specialist cover, education and training, and on consultant work patterns; as well as the impact of Modernising Medical Careers on the design of training programmes in renal medicine

▶ the changing roles of other professional groups within the renal multiprofessional team, for example expansion in nurse consultants and nurse specialists, and the implications of extended prescribing.

1.2   The pattern of day-to-day clinical work for renal physicians is also in flux. Relevant influences include:

▶ the increasing need for care of patients with end-stage renal disease (ESRD) and the increasing age of the ESRD population

▶ the increasing role for renal physicians in the long-term care of transplant recipients away from RTUs

▶ the decreasing involvement of renal physicians in the care of patients with acute renal failure in intensive care units

- ▶ the increasing role of radiologists in renal biopsy and other interventional work for renal patients

- ▶ the increasing emphasis on early detection and management of chronic kidney disease requiring new integrated ways of working with primary care and other areas of secondary care

- ▶ the importance of effective transfer of young people from paediatric care, a time of high clinical risk.

While renal medicine remains a relatively popular specialty with few unfilled consultant posts, circumstances are changing. Both consultant and specialty registrar posts, often attract a small number of applicants. Renal medicine was associated with a long hours culture which was the basis of its original success when it was a fledgling specialty building the notion of holistic care for people with complex chronic illness. In the changing environment this is a disincentive for recruitment, particularly of women.

1.3   The Royal College of Physicians is very active in discussion with the Department of Health and the training authorities about the broad impact of some of these changes on the future role of consultant physicians. However, rapid changes in the organisation and practice of renal medicine mean that the specialty requires specific analysis and specific proposals. A number of particular groups within the renal medicine medical workforce have issues requiring review – for example women in renal medicine and non-consultant career grades. However, rather than dealing with any of these groups individually, this Working Party has reviewed these issues in an integrated way, analysing the implications for the whole medical workforce in renal medicine.

Patient perspective

1.4   Renal patients would like a patient-centred, holistic approach to their care. They wish for a choice of modality of renal replacement therapy, together with support from all members of the multiprofessional renal team.

Remit

1.5   The Working Party investigated the impact of all the factors described above on all groups within the renal medicine medical workforce including:

- ▶ NHS consultants

- ▶ clinical academics

- ▶ specialty registrars

- ▶ staff grades and associate specialists

- ▶ medical specialties with clinical links to renal medicine

- ▶ representatives of the multiprofessional renal team.

Representatives of patients and commissioners were also consulted.

In this report, the Working Party makes recommendations relevant to the current practice of renal medicine and its development as a specialty over the next eight to ten years.

The Working Party recognises that many of the challenges in providing specialist medical services and acute general medicine are common to all medical specialties. For this reason we consider that a proportion of our recommendations will have relevance to other medical specialties.

The final draft of this report was prepared after all witnesses and stakeholders had had an opportunity to review a detailed draft of the whole document.

2 Provision of renal services in the UK

The historical development of renal services in the UK

2.1   In the 1970s and 1980s, renal units developed in teaching hospitals, with links to universities. Undergraduate and postgraduate training occurred predominantly in these university teaching hospitals. Since the 1990s most new renal units have developed in DGHs, with the objective of not only increasing capacity, but also bringing renal services closer to the patients. In addition, the DGHs now make a greater contribution to both undergraduate and postgraduate education as some have acquired teaching hospital status or become the site of new medical schools. Therefore the renal services in these two types of hospitals are broadly similar, with the exception that renal transplantation usually takes place in the traditional university teaching hospitals. For the purpose of this report, the Working Party has designated a renal unit as either an RTU or an RU.

Renal services in the UK: the current position

2.2   Renal physicians investigate, treat and follow up patients with a wide range of renal disease in both inpatient and outpatient settings. Some of these patients develop progressive CKD, leading to established renal failure requiring renal replacement therapy by dialysis or renal transplantation.

2.3   The *Eighth Annual Report* of the UK Renal Registry (December 2005) reports that there are around 140,000 CKD patients under the care of renal physicians in UK renal units, of whom around 23,000 have advanced CKD (stage 4 and 5), although not yet requiring renal replacement therapy.[1] These CKD patients are managed in outpatient clinics of hospitals with renal units or in satellite renal clinics in other DGHs. Many CKD patients are also under shared care with primary care, and with other secondary care specialists.

2.4   There are 73 renal units in England and Wales, Scotland and Northern Ireland. These units look after more than 38,000 renal replacement therapy patients. Over 20,000 patients are on dialysis; 74% on haemodialysis and 26% on peritoneal dialysis (PD). Over 18,000 patients have functioning renal transplants. Most patients receive haemodialysis in the main hospital renal unit, but increasingly also in satellite haemodialysis units. A small proportion of patients still undertake home haemodialysis. A satellite unit is a dialysis unit whose organisation and governance is provided by an NHS renal unit and whose dialysis activities are protocol driven within an NHS-managed clinical network. Satellite units are sited in other DGHs or in community dialysis facilities, in order to be nearer patients' homes. Over the past 20 years some satellite units have been built and equipped by private providers and others by the NHS within these governance arrangements, allowing a seamless integrated care pathway for NHS patients.

2.5   In 2004 the estimated adult acceptance rate for renal replacement therapy in the UK was 103 new patients per million population (pmp), with 6,088 patients commencing renal replacement therapy. In addition, 104 children started renal replacement therapy. The established modality of dialysis after 90 days of renal replacement therapy was haemodialysis in 73% of patients and peritoneal dialysis in 24%. In 2004, only 3% of those commencing had received a transplant as a primary modality. The minimum estimated prevalence of renal replacement therapy in the UK at the end of 2003 was 638 pmp. The local authority prevalence varied considerably from 322 to 1,108 pmp. There has been an annual increase in prevalence in the 27 English and Welsh units participating in the UK Renal Registry since 2002 of around 5%.

2.6   The prevalence of renal replacement therapy rises with age, the largest prevalence being 1,837 pmp in men between 80 and 85 years. Consequently the age of patients on HD is increasing; 22% of new patients starting renal replacement therapy, and 12% of all patients on renal replacement therapy are 75 years or older. An increasing number of patients do not wish for dialysis treatment or are considered medically unsuitable for dialysis as a result of co-morbid conditions. They are managed with non-dialysis care.

2.7   Renal units also provide investigative and treatment facilities, including dialysis for patients with acute renal failure. Such patients may be transferred from smaller DGHs without renal units to RTUs and RUs. Patients with multi-organ failure are jointly managed by renal physicians and critical care physicians on critical care units, while more stable patients with acute renal failure will be managed by renal physicians on renal wards, sometimes in a designated renal high dependency unit.

2.8   Four models of provision of renal services have emerged:

- ▶ RTUs, typically with six to ten consultant renal physicians, providing a visiting service for surrounding DGHs

- ▶ RUs in teaching hospitals or larger DGHs, typically with three to six renal physicians who might also provide a visiting renal service to smaller neighbouring DGHs

- ▶ Units with only one or two renal physicians providing a full renal service with a 1:1 or 1:2 on-call rota for renal medicine

- ▶ Single-handed renal physicians in hospitals providing a 9am to 5pm service and on call for renal medicine when on call for general medicine. These hospitals work in conjunction with an RTU which provides outs-of-hours cover.

2.9   Renal transplants are performed in RTUs. In recent years there has been a trend for potential transplant recipients and living donors to receive an increasing proportion of the pre-transplant evaluation in RUs. In addition, patients with functioning transplants are increasingly being referred back to RUs, in some units immediately after the postoperative period. Staffing, both medical and nursing, in RUs needs to reflect the growing number of transplant patients under follow-up in these units.

2.10   Renal physicians work in close association with multiprofessional health workers, particularly nurses, pharmacists, dieticians, psychologists and social workers. Care of renal patients also involves liaison with other specialties such as diabetes, vascular access surgery, paediatrics and palliative care, as well as with local kidney patient associations. In addition, patients with acute renal failure in the setting of multi-organ failure are usually jointly managed with critical care physicians and anaesthetists.

Renal units

2.11   Much of the expansion of renal services in the UK has been in RUs – mostly in DGHs – although some are in teaching hospitals, where another teaching hospital provides the RTU. The majority of renal physicians in RUs also participate in the acute medical on-call rota, although some have reduced their commitment compared with other medical specialties. GIM accounts for 30–50% of the workload of renal physicians in RUs, which serve smaller populations than traditional teaching centres: commonly at least 0.5 million population. RUs typically have a poorer infrastructure than RTUs, and fewer medical staff, both at career grades and training grades. Despite this, both postgraduate and undergraduate teaching commitments are often similar. It is a view in some DGHs that the opening of satellite haemodialysis units has delayed or prevented appropriate development of an RU. On the other hand, in some instances, the setting up of a satellite unit has given impetus to the development of an RU.

Regional variations

2.12   In Scotland, allocation of health funding per capita is 10–15% greater than in England and Wales. The prevalence of renal replacement therapy is also higher in Scotland than in England and Wales, being approximately 800 pmp. The RTUs are situated in the university centres of Glasgow and Edinburgh. As well as two RTUs in Scotland there are seven RUs. Reorganisation of renal services is ongoing, concentrating specialist services in the major centres. For example in Glasgow in 1999, three teaching hospital trusts offered inpatient renal services. By 2004 inpatient services had been concentrated in two hospitals, and future plans are that inpatient facilities will concentrate in one Glasgow hospital supplemented by facilities in two ambulatory care and diagnostic centres, with a satellite dialysis unit in 9 of the 12 local hospitals.

2.13   In Northern Ireland there is one RTU in Belfast with five RUs in DGHs with mixed models of out-of-hours service provision. The nephrologist in the RU within the greater Belfast area contributes to the RTU's on-call rota. The nephrologists in Antrim provide 50% of the local out-of-hours nephrology cover, with the remaining 50% provided by the RTU. In the more remote south-east and west of Northern Ireland, out-of-hours cover is provided by the local physicians and nephrologists. The local nephrologists operate as a network to cover both RUs in the west. The RTU provides out-of-hours cover for other acute hospitals without on-site renal units and can take appropriate complex cases from RUs at any time. The RUs have traditionally been staffed by single-handed nephrologists. Consultant recruitment has been problematic, affected by such factors as salary differentials with the Republic of Ireland. The strength of the renal services in Northern Ireland has been planning future capacity with the active involvement of the Chief Medical Officer, though there is now considerable uncertainty surrounding the future of commissioning.

2.14   The strength of provision of renal services in Northern Ireland is helped by an integrated commissioning process and in Scotland by greater funding. There are greater inequalities of provision of renal services in England and Wales; in Wales there are separate commissioning arrangements. In the 57 renal units in England and Wales, there is a wide variation in numbers of renal replacement therapy patients, from 68 to 1,398 patients. In the larger, long-established RTUs up to 67% of renal replacement therapy patients have a functioning transplant whereas in RUs, with usually between 200 and 800 renal replacement therapy patients only 25–50% will have a functioning transplant. The expansion of renal services in England and Wales over the past few years has been increasingly in DGHs with the establishment or expansion of RUs in these hospitals. Such units often perceive that local commissioners and NHS trusts lack understanding of the requirements for staffing and infrastructure of a renal unit.

RECOMMENDATIONS

We recommend two preferred models for renal units: either a renal and transplant unit (RTU) providing a visiting service for surrounding DGHs, or a renal unit (RU) which might also provide a visiting service to smaller neighbouring DGHs. A population of 0.5 million is typically sufficient to justify the need for an RU, although local geographical factors might influence the size of population served.

We recommend that there should be little distinction made between RUs (usually in DGHs) and RTUs in the traditional teaching hospitals, in the range of services provided, other than acute transplantation. In addition, there should be no distinction in the need for supporting services (for example surgery, imaging and laboratory services) nor in the staffing requirements in the renal unit of both career grades and training grades of medical staff and other health professionals.

3 Medical staffing of renal units

Consultants

3.1   The Royal College of Physicians consultant census, 2005, showed that there were 359 consultant renal physicians in the UK.[2] Of these, 289 were consultants in England, 13 in Wales, 10 in Northern Ireland and 47 in Scotland. Between 2004 and 2005 there was a 3.2% increase in consultants in England.[2,3] Less than 10% of consultants had academic or research contracts.

3.2   Renal medicine is generally perceived to be a high intensity specialty with a long hours ethos which has been exacerbated for consultants by a reduction in junior doctor hours as a result of the EWTD. The Royal College of Physicians consultant census, 2005 showed that renal physicians worked on average 56 hours per week, and that 41% of them exceeded 48 working hours per week. Working hours for consultant renal physicians are among the highest of all medical specialties. Based on 2006 service levels, a 49% increase in consultant renal physicians would be necessary to enable existing consultants to meet the requirements of EWTD.

3.3   Most consultants in RTUs no longer participate in the on-call rotas for unselected medical emergency admissions, while in RUs the majority of consultants still participate in such rotas, and also take responsibility for continuing care of GIM patients. The 2005 census identified that 51.4% of renal physicians have a GIM commitment. Most renal physicians in RUs consider that participation in general medicine is an important part of their professional role, particularly as DGHs provide training opportunities in GIM for specialty registrars. Nevertheless consultants, with 30% to 50% of their present workload related to GIM, are increasingly reducing or considering withdrawing from their commitment to GIM as renal medicine workloads continue to increase.

3.4   We recommend that a minimum of four renal physicians is required to provide a satisfactory on-call renal rota. A minimum of two consultant appointments is necessary to establish a new renal unit, and a minimum of four consultants is required before a renal unit becomes autonomous in providing all services other than acute transplantation. Autonomy should usually be attained within five years and during that interim period, the units should be supported by a managed clinical network. There are presently 16 renal units with less than four renal physicians: six in England, two in Wales, four in Northern Ireland and four in Scotland. New renal units are still being established with single-handed renal physicians and insecure plans from hospital trusts and commissioners for consultant expansion. There are a few single-handed renal physicians who are still providing renal medicine services but without chronic dialysis facilities.

3.5   It is generally agreed that between eight and ten renal StRs are needed to provide a full shift on-call renal rota, but these numbers of StRs are not available in RUs, nor in a number of RTUs. The increasing use of 'Hospital at Night' and other services assumes that non-specialised staff can provide optimal night cover for renal wards. However, the replacement of on-call rotas for specialty registrars in renal medicine by such means is often inappropriate for the specific needs of patients with complex renal disease. For RUs, this situation currently represents an impasse which can only be addressed by very substantial investment in numbers of doctors working in these units.

3.6   The National Renal Workforce Planning Group, under the auspices of the Royal College of Nursing, the Royal College of Physicians and the Royal College of Paediatrics and Child Health, published in 2002 *The renal team: a multiprofessional renal workforce plan for adults and children with renal disease.*[4] This report noted that the 2001 establishment of renal physicians was 290. The requirement in 2001 was calculated as 512, with the requirement in 2010 increasing to 803. The calculation of consultant numbers is based on the duties of renal physicians and their various roles and responsibilities as described in the document *Consultant physicians working with patients* (3rd edition, 2004).[5] This suggests one consultant renal physician per 75 renal replacement therapy patients or one whole-time equivalent (WTE) per 100 renal replacement therapy patients. This figure could underestimate the actual requirement taking account of GIM responsibilities and the reduced number of doctors in training in RUs. Case mix influences the appropriate workload. For example, if a consultant's major responsibility is the care of patients with established renal transplants rather than dialysis patients, a higher number of patients per consultant is appropriate.

3.7   In common with many other medical specialties, renal physicians increasingly provide specialist advice by telephone, letter or electronic communication. This important and increasing component of consultant work should be recognised in the job planning process.

3.8   In order to optimise use of consultant time, it is essential that trusts continue to provide them with sufficient personal assistant support. This recognises the various and simultaneous responsibilities consultants currently fulfil.

3.9   The present number of trainees in renal medicine will not support the expansion of consultant numbers required. In the next 10 years, 30% of renal physicians will retire, and approximately 2% per annum take up appointments in non-clinical management or industry.

RECOMMENDATIONS

We recommend that there should be a substantial increase in the number of consultant renal physicians in the UK, particularly in RUs with a GIM commitment. This should include positive support for consultants wishing to work flexibly. We recommend that one consultant renal physician is required per 75 renal replacement therapy patients or one WTE per 100 renal replacement therapy patients. If a consultant is responsible for the care of patients with established renal transplants, a higher number of patients per consultant is appropriate. These figures could underestimate the requirement in RUs where consultants have a major commitment to GIM and where there are usually fewer specialty registrars.

We recommend that a minimum of two consultant appointments is necessary to establish a new renal unit, and a minimum of four consultants is required before a renal unit can be autonomous and provide all services other than acute transplantation. Autonomy should usually be attained within five years and during the interim period the unit should be supported by a managed clinical network.

We recommend that a commitment to GIM should not be expected to continue throughout a consultant career. The career development of individuals may result in their taking over other responsibilities such as management and teaching, and in changes in their clinical commitments including GIM.

Staff grades and associate specialists

3.10   Staff grades and associate specialists make an important contribution to the provision of renal care in the UK. A census by the Renal Association in 2004 indicated that there were 66 doctors in these positions working in UK renal units; 34 being staff grades, 27 associate specialists, four clinical assistants and one trust grade doctor. In another survey in 2002, 81% had postgraduate qualifications and worked an average of 9.3 sessions. The majority worked on dialysis units; commitment to inpatient renal medicine was variable and few had any commitment to GIM. Nearly half (46%) had no on-call commitment and 44% were involved in a renal on-call rota, mostly at middle-grade level. Of these staff, 67% expressed the wish to join the Specialist Register and thus be eligible for consultant posts, which might be possible under the regulations of the PMETB.[6]

3.11   Entry to the Specialist Register is now possible via article 14 of PMETB, for doctors who can demonstrate the equivalence of training and requisite experience. PMETB has charged the Joint Committee on Higher Medical Training (JCHMT) with assessing applications, and this will be accomplished by renal Specialist Advisory Committee (SAC) of the Royal College of Physicians members (and others as regional specialty advisors) who have been trained in Article 14 assessment. This entry route is available to both UK and overseas graduates. However, the application of these regulations might disadvantage those who have only worked in the UK, and prevent them from being eligible for the Specialist Register.

3.12   While staff grades and associate specialists in renal medicine often do not have training and experience consistent with the broad role of a consultant nephrologist, many have high-grade specialist expertise in aspects of renal medicine, most commonly dialysis medicine.

RECOMMENDATIONS

We recommend that staff grades and associates specialists should be actively encouraged to join the Specialist Register, if necessary re-entering specialty training to do so. Flexible training should be available to facilitate such career development.

We recommend that there is clarification of entry to the Specialist Register via Article 14 of the PMETB for doctors trained solely in the UK, who might currently be excluded from the Specialist Register under these regulations.

We recommend that dialysis medicine becomes an approved specialty to which PMETB can offer specialist registration

Specialty registrars in renal medicine and general internal medicine

Structure, organisation and monitoring of specialty registrar training

3.13   The SAC of the Royal College of Physicians oversees the training of StRs, writes the renal curriculum, and ensures its proper delivery by training programmes, as well as approving completion of training. It also has an input into workforce planning, and works with postgraduate deans to ensure that the national training numbers awarded by the Workforce Review Team are funded, and are translated into educationally approved training posts. There is some uncertainty regarding the complexity of the workforce planning process which presently involves not only SACs but also deaneries, the Department of Health Workforce Review Team, PMETB, regional speciality advisors and local training committees. There is particular concern that the SAC will no longer undertake visits to assess specialty training programmes; this responsibility has devolved to PMETB whose deanery-wide visits may not be able to assess individual specialty training programmes in the same detail that was previously achieved by SAC visits.

3.14   In 2005, 27 new National Training Numbers (NTN) were allocated, but only 22 bids had been received for training posts; local funding issues are the major block since funding clinical services is often prioritised above funding for StR training. In recent years the Workforce Review Team has received representation for the creation of 64 new posts per annum. Although a smaller number of posts have eventually been approved (between 20 and 40 per annum), it has not always been possible to create these in practice, primarily because of funding issues.

3.15   There is a potential conflict between training opportunities for StRs and their clinical responsibilities.

3.16   The reforms proposed in Modernising Medical Careers are not a direct responsibility of the SAC but have implications for entry into training in the specialty.[7] There remains uncertainty as to the stage at which a trainee should choose the higher training specialty to pursue; the second year of core medical training seems the most likely. Having to make a decision about a career at an earlier stage might deny trainees sufficient time and opportunities to sample different aspects of medicine, particularly in smaller specialties such as renal medicine to which there may be less exposure in medical school or in foundation year posts. If training times are to be compressed then the renal curriculum would have to be fashioned with shortened periods of training, making out-of-programme experience for research or other additional training opportunities more difficult to arrange. Additional specialty training, for example in transplant medicine, might be deferred until after completion of the renal medicine curriculum.

Specialty training

3.17   In April 2005, the JCHMT database identified 301 SpRs (now termed StRs) undergoing training in renal medicine and GIM. The proportion of female trainees (37%) was identical to respiratory medicine, similar to endocrinology and diabetes (40%) but higher than cardiology (19%) and gastroenterology (24%). By February 2006 the total number of renal trainees had increased to 329. Only seven SpRs were training flexibly, of whom six were women. Currently the majority of medical undergraduates are women. Renal medicine may become less popular with female graduates if there are few opportunities for flexible training within SpR rotations.

3.18   A questionnaire was sent by the Education and Training Committee of the Renal Association in 2003 to all renal medicine training committees and to SpRs, with a response rate of 33%. This indicated that 80% of trainees were intending to dually accredit in renal medicine and GIM, although the number of SpRs intending not to dual accredit or not apply for consultant posts which include a general medical commitment is increasing. A questionnaire circulated by the JCHMT in December 2004 resulted in replies from 47 renal medicine SpRs (16%), of whom only 64% wished to continue doing acute general medical take.[8] Consultant appointments in RUs and particularly in smaller hospitals were less popular, with only 11% of SpRs aiming to obtain a DGH consultant appointment, although 21% were undecided. There is uncertainty about the impact of Modernising Medical Careers on dual accreditation in renal medicine and general medicine.

3.19   Doctors in training perceive renal medicine to be an intensive specialty with long hours. The number of applications for SpR posts has diminished in recent years, with an average of 5.5 applicants per post, and 3.5 candidates being shortlisted.

3.20   Experiential learning in renal medicine during training has reduced in recent years. SpRs express concerns that changes in on-call rotas, including shift working, result in a lack of continuity and reduce the amount of quality time spent at work. If trainees are required to work a full-shift rota, it has been estimated in one training programme that there will be a reduction of outpatient clinic experience from 260 clinics to 137 in four years of training. Analysis of an SpR diary showed that as a result of EWTD, there has been a 50% reduction in overall exposure to renal training opportunities. Participation in medical on-call rotas in RUs reduces experiences in renal medicine in those hospitals.

3.21   While experiential training should remain an integral part of training, the flexibility required to run such a system has an impact on delivery of clinical services. The reduction in trainee involvement in clinics requires more work from consultants over and above agreed programmed activities. Competency training is time consuming for both trainees and trainers.

3.22   The curriculum for renal medicine is self-contained; it has been developed by the SAC, and is delivered within units and through educational programmes run by training committees supported by appropriate national educational initiatives (for example the annual Advanced Nephrology Course of the Renal Association). There may be opportunities to develop modular elements within the curriculum which can be made available to trainees in other specialties, with similar access for renal medicine trainees to relevant modules in other specialty training programmes, for example in diabetes and cardiology.

3.23   Following completion of training in renal medicine, further experience over and above the renal medicine curriculum may need to be undertaken to ensure the expertise of the future consultant workforce to deliver the clinical service. Specialised areas may include dialysis medicine, interventional nephrology, critical care nephrology and transplant medicine.

3.24   At any time, about 20% of renal medicine trainees are doing research. This varies between deaneries; in some deaneries, less than half the trainees had any research opportunities. Undertaking research during clinical posts can be challenging because of pressure of clinical commitments. Some SpRs report difficulty in finding funding to carry out research, or to develop an academic career.

3.25   While it is not necessary for all trainees to take time out for research, some experience of research during clinical posts, or training in research methodology, is necessary for professional development. Doctors in training should be encouraged to develop aspects of their professional work in addition to clinical training which will contribute positively to their future career. As well as research, other suitable expertise includes education, management and information technology.

RECOMMENDATIONS

We recommend that interest in renal medicine as a career is encouraged early in training by ensuring that medical students have a positive experience of the specialty during their undergraduate training, and then by offering experience in renal medicine during the foundation years.

We recommend that the process of organisation and monitoring of specialty training is streamlined, with clearer description of the responsibilities of the involved organisations.

We recommend that local funding issues should not delay the establishment of specialty training posts which have received workforce and educational approval.

We recommend that opportunities for flexible training for doctors in training are expanded, are part of mainstream service provision and are readily funded.

We recommend that competency-based training is developed to complement (but not replace) experiential learning, with sufficient resources for postgraduate medical education including the increased availability of web-based distance learning, to ensure that support for competency-based training does not compromise patient care.

We recommend that opportunities be developed to share modules of training with other specialties, for example diabetes and cardiology.

We recommend that there should be opportunities after completion of renal medical training for additional experience enabling renal physicians to develop accredited subspecialty expertise in dialysis medicine, critical care nephrology, interventional nephrology, and transplant medicine.

Academic renal medicine

3.26   A series of reports have documented the decline of clinical academic medicine in the UK in the past decade.[9–13] Data published by the Council of Heads of Medical Schools show that in 2000, clinical academics made up 8% of the total NHS consultant workforce; in 2004 this had decreased to 6.5%.[14] Of particular concern is the decline in the number of clinical lecturers, which in 2004 stood at 58% of the 2000 figures.

3.27   The *Walport Report* set out a series of recommendations to reverse these trends.[15] These address the key stages of a clinician's career namely medical school, foundation training, specialty training and consultant grade. Within specialty training it is recommended that clinical fellowships and clinical lectureships are established to provide a dedicated academic training programme. After specialty training, it is recommended that new clinical senior lectureships are established to augment currently available academic training programmes across England and Wales.

3.28   In 2006, the implementation of these recommendations saw the appointment of the first cadre of clinical fellows, clinical lecturers and clinical senior lecturers. These programmes form part of the new national health research strategy Best Research for Best Health.[16] Other key features of this strategy are the establishment of a National Institute for Health Research in England (**www.nihr.ac.uk**), the establishment of a Clinical Research Network (**www.ukcrn.org.uk/index.html**) and an expansion of NHS investment in clinical research facilities. Underpinning this is the UK clinical research collaboration (**www.ukcrc.org**) which brings together the major stakeholders influencing clinical research in the UK to establish '*a partnership working to establish the UK as a world leader in clinical research, by harnessing the power of the NHS*'. Renal medicine is well placed to take advantage of the opportunities offered by a clinical research network. The coherence of the specialty, the close clinical and academic working relationships among renal units and the high level of research training characteristic of consultants all contribute to a research infrastructure with great potential.

3.29   Renal medicine has a very strong academic tradition. The Renal Association was initially founded in 1950 as a scientific society, and although now involved in all aspects of clinical renal medicine, it maintains its strong focus on education and research. The first renal units to be established in the UK were all attached to academic departments.

3.30   Exposure to research during specialty training continues to be encouraged. Traditionally trainees have undertaken a formal period of research resulting in a higher degree (Masters degree or PhD). In the future this may not be appropriate for all trainees, with some undertaking a shorter period of research resulting in a Masters degree and others choosing to gain additional experience in education or management.

3.31   The limited funding available for research and the inflexibility of training programmes are seen as significant deterrents to trainees considering an academic career. The opportunities for research training vary from region to region. Competition for national research training fellowships is intense and in some areas the availability of local funding is limited. The mechanism by which the Walport clinical fellowships and lectureships will be assimilated into renal medicine training programmes is not clear. There is concern that academic renal medicine might not benefit from this new scheme because it is perceived already to be relatively strong. Experience from the Medical Research Council, the Wellcome Trust and medical charities, suggest there is no shortage of potential clinical academics who intend to specialise in renal medicine applying for training fellowships.

3.32   The contribution of established academic renal physicians to the local clinical programme is variable. In some regions it is felt that the clinical workload undertaken by clinical academics is excessive. A split of at least 50% academic:50% clinical is considered by many to be an appropriate balance. The clinical training of clinical academics should be of an equivalent standard to their full-time clinical counterparts. However, many clinical academics choose to train only in renal medicine, and not in GIM.

3.33   There are also considerable opportunities for renal units to participate in programmes of research and development with immediate clinical applicability. Such programmes might involve many renal healthcare workers, for example in the development of dialysis technology or evaluation of new models of clinical care. Experience in cancer networks has shown the benefit to clinical care of increased recruitment of patients into clinical trials. In renal medicine, development in research will benefit patients by refining treatment of renal diseases, for example improving transplant immunosuppressive regimens.

RECOMMENDATIONS

We recommend that trainees are given the opportunity to undertake original research with the aim of achieving a higher degree during specialty training. We recognise that full-time research will not be undertaken by all trainees, but all should have exposure to research methodology. We recommend that trainees also avail themselves of opportunities to develop experience in other aspects of professional work including education and management.

We recommend that there should be opportunities to undertake such training on a flexible basis.

We recommend that a split of 50% academic:50% clinical is an appropriate balance in workload for academic nephrologists.

We recommend the establishment of a UK clinical research network in renal disease.

4 Provision of patient-centred care

The patient perspective

4.1 Patient groups welcomed the National Service Framework (NSF) for Renal Services for England, but were concerned that this was more of a mission statement rather than a detailed implementation plan.[17,18] Patients look to a national vision for a patient-centred service. Renal patients have identified the need for:

- ▶ a holistic approach to their care from renal healthcare workers, treating the patient not the disease

- ▶ meeting cultural needs and providing emotional support

- ▶ medicines management with advice and information

- ▶ training

- ▶ adequate staff communication

- ▶ dietary advice

- ▶ integrated care plans

- ▶ opportunities for dialysis away from home

- ▶ assistance with financial benefits

- ▶ availability of counselling services

- ▶ ability to maintain employment

- ▶ an appropriate environment in renal units

- ▶ patient choice, involving choice of modality, time of dialysis and when and where to die

- ▶ adequate transport to renal units, with accepted national guidelines for provision of transportation and reimbursement of costs.

4.2 Patients have expressed concern that inadequate staffing of renal units may limit opportunities for patients to see a consultant regularly and that the consultant workload is sometimes too onerous to allow sufficient listening time. Staff attitudes can appear, on occasion, uncaring due to work pressures. Patients recognise that it is not always possible to see their own consultant, but they consider that the doctors should be aware of their condition and circumstances and should liaise with other healthcare professionals involved in their care. This can be difficult to achieve in larger, busier hospitals where patients may prefer to deal with nursing staff, who are sometimes perceived as having more time and sympathy. Changes in junior doctors' working practices are not seen to be a major issue with regard to reducing continuity of care, but problems may be experienced in accessing medical staff in satellite units.

4.3   Despite these concerns the majority of renal patients expressed satisfaction with their medical care. Although dialysis capacity has improved over the past few years, there are still concerns that renal units are working at 100% capacity, as a result of staffing issues and resources. Patients are often unable to dialyse at units close to home or have to dialyse at inconvenient times of day. There is concern from patient groups that some patients, particularly older patients, might not be offered dialysis because of capacity issues. Patients remain concerned about inadequate provision of vascular access for haemodialysis. Late referral of patients to renal units is one factor, but there are still significant problems with capacity for vascular access surgery, and organisation of services.

4.4   Patients have expressed concern that less than half of renal patients have a documented care plan. Renal healthcare workers should work together with patients to develop such treatment plans. The need for psychological support is regarded by patients to be extremely important since it covers most of the personal, family, financial, employment and social aspects of patient lifestyle. Availability of support from psychologists varies widely between renal units. Social work support for renal patients is typically below national standards. Where dedicated renal social workers are available they are not infrequently funded from charitable sources. The 1991 Workforce Recommendations indicated that, for example, a unit with 200 dialysis patients and 600 transplant and pre-dialysis patients should have three WTE social workers.[19] Fifteen years later, this requirement is still unmet.

4.5   Arrangements for funding for temporary dialysis away from home are suboptimal. In the UK, NHS trusts are responsible for the cost of patients undergoing dialysis away from home within the UK, whereas for dialysis in other EU countries there is central funding available. The minimum entitlement of 12 dialysis treatments per annum recommended by the Department of Health is not always available.

4.6   In summary, patients feel that the largest barriers to choice in their treatment are capacity and resource issues. Patients have concerns that funding intended for specific renal specialised services may be diverted to other priorities in primary care trusts. Therefore, an integrated approach to commissioning for specialised services is necessary.

The development of renal replacement therapy services

4.7   Appropriate choice of modality of renal replacement therapy is an important element of renal care. For some patients, the optimum mode of renal replacement therapy will be influenced by medical considerations. Haemodialysis is offered in dialysis units in RTUs and RUs. More stable patients may be able to dialyse in satellite dialysis units, which ideally are closer to the patient's home. There may be opportunities to establish satellite units near or within primary care health centres, or in other community settings. However, pressure on dialysis capacity means that it is not possible for all patients to dialyse in the most geographically convenient dialysis unit. The National Institute for Health and Clinical Excellence (NICE) guideline for home haemodialysis recommends that home haemodialysis should be offered to those patients who desire this mode of treatment and are medically suitable.[20] Peritoneal dialysis may be offered to patients either in the form of continuous ambulatory peritoneal dialysis (CAPD), or as machine-operated automated peritoneal dialysis (APD). Many patients will be considered suitable for renal transplantation. While most patients will receive a well-matched kidney from a deceased donor, receiving a kidney from a living donor reduces the waiting time for a suitably matched kidney, and also has benefits of better transplant survival. In some patients, other diseases, particularly cardiovascular disease, increase the risk of morbidity and mortality related to transplantation so that remaining on dialysis improves survival.

Vascular access surgery

4.8   Availability of vascular access surgery remains a major concern in most renal units, as highlighted by the UK Dialysis Access Survey 2005.[1] The opportunity for patients to have arteriovenous fistulae and grafts performed without delay can be restricted by a range of deficiencies in the care pathway including delay in surgical referral, lack of vascular surgeons, lack of outpatient clinic capacity and lack of operating theatre time. Hospitals often prioritise routine waiting list operations ahead of vascular access. Comparative data with Europe show increased usage of percutaneous dialysis catheters in the UK.[21] Catheter use is associated with increased morbidity and mortality, including healthcare-acquired infection. A report of a project commissioned by the Department of Health at two sites was published in 2005 and sets out the pathways to improve availability of vascular access surgery to patients.[22]

RECOMMENDATION

We recommend that renal services are developed in line with the standards and markers of good practice in the National Service Framework for Renal Services for England and equivalent framework documents in other parts of the UK; ensuring that patient-centred, holistic care is available for all renal patients.

The multiprofessional renal team

4.9   The management of renal patients requires the collaboration of a number of professional groups, including nurses, dieticians, pharmacists, social workers, clinical psychologists, technicians and healthcare assistants, each with unique and essential contributions to holistic patient care. These professional groups are increasingly undertaking extended roles, and many of the traditional duties of the medical staff are now being satisfactorily performed by other professional groups. Such a structure has considerable advantages since improved accessibility and focused working can enhance patient care and the patient experience. This gives opportunities for the role of renal physicians within the multiprofessional team to be refined to ensure the best use of medical expertise and experience.

Nursing

4.10   The skill-mix required within renal nursing is described in *The renal team: a multi-professional renal workforce plan (recommendations of the National Renal Workforce Planning Group, 2002).*[4] There is a shortfall in nursing which is not unique to renal services. International recruitment has made a valuable contribution but this may have reached its peak.

4.11   Enhanced roles for nurses in renal care are long established. Wide clinical responsibility and independent decision making have characterised the work of nurses in dialysis units for 30 years.

4.12   Nursing roles are now being extended further into nurse practitioner and nurse consultant appointments. Developments in non-medical prescribing offer further opportunities to develop enhanced roles, particularly related to anaemia management, bone disease, hypertension control and dialysis adequacy.

4.13   The 2004/05 Renal Workforce Competency Framework describes the activities needed to deliver care to patients as well as the standards required.[23] Nine areas related to dialysis were completed and covered all healthcare professionals including nursing staff. Areas of renal competence that are developed or under development are: renal replacement, renal management, renal life, awaiting transplant, living donor, deceased donation, transplantation operation, transplanted patient and ongoing processes. This should help to create a workforce flexible enough to respond to new demands, but support will be required from medical and other staff as these new roles develop. The individual patient's needs remain paramount.

4.14   Nurse consultant and advanced nurse practitioner roles are being developed in order to enhance the quality of patient care and may reduce the impact of changes to junior doctors' working hours. Nurses may support the work of medical staff as nurse consultants and advanced practitioners through Hospital at Night initiatives and supplementary prescribing, working within medically approved care pathways.

4.15   There are opportunities for developing nurse roles including transplant liaison, diabetes/renal nurse specialist, anaemia nurse specialist, live donor coordinator, dialysis access coordinator and discharge coordinator. A few nurses have been trained as surgical assistants for the insertion of percutaneous tunnelled lines for dialysis.

4.16   There are also opportunities for developing renal nursing expertise in primary care, particularly in the management of CKD. For instance, community matrons and long-term condition case managers can use skills in renal nursing, cardiovascular disease and diabetes to develop tools for screening, surveillance and education in patients with CKD associated vascular diseases.

Healthcare assistants

4.17   Healthcare assistants have had a long-standing role in supporting nurses in the haemodialysis units and on renal wards. As nurses take on extended roles there are opportunities for healthcare assistants to develop new skills and take over more areas of renal nursing, particularly on dialysis units. The development of the National Workforce Competency Framework should facilitate the development of skills for groups such as healthcare assistants.[24]

Pharmacists

4.18   With patients on multiple and complex medication regimens, there is the necessity for robust communication with primary care about changes to medication. Medicines management facilitates optimum care at all stages. Around 10% of medicines are not taken by patients as prescribed, for a variety of reasons including poor communication. This accounts for a significant number of hospital admissions. Pharmacists have participated in anaemia management in renal patients in some hospitals. Pharmacists could undertake systematic medicine reviews with patients to facilitate understanding, and liaise with community pharmacists for patients managed by shared care with primary care. Electronic patient records will facilitate prescribing and communication between primary and secondary care.

Dieticians

4.19   The recent NICE recommendations have emphasised the importance of nutrition on patients' quality of life.[24] Dieticians play an important role in identifying and managing nutritional problems and in diabetes management. In conjunction with physicians, they can develop roles in monitoring and alteration of medication related to renal bone disease.

Clinical psychologists

4.20   Psychological assessment and support help patients adapt to dialysis and improve quality of life. Psychological support as part of a multiprofessional team can succeed in increasing the number of patients participating in their therapies. Psychologists may identify problems that have not been revealed to doctors and nurses. Psychological assessment is helpful, and in some cases necessary, in the work-up of patients being considered as potential transplant recipients.

Social workers

4.21   Social work input to renal patients facilitates the transfer of care to the community. Assistance with home support, aids and advice empower renal patients and increase the likelihood of patients keeping to their treatment regimens. Social workers can identify patient problems in the community which can be communicated to medical and nursing staff

Workforce planning

4.22   The National Renal Workforce Planning Group recommended the workforce requirements at the time of the report (2001) and requirements by 2010.[4]

RECOMMENDATIONS

We recommend the continuing expansion of competency-based training for all health professionals in the renal multiprofessional team, allowing extended roles for nurses and other practitioners.

We recommend redefining the roles of doctors within the renal multiprofessional team wherever this is appropriate to the holistic care of patients and the professional development of other members of the team. A goal of this redefinition is to allow the most effective use of the specific skills of physicians in evaluation, diagnosis and overall responsibility for patient management.

Transplant medicine

4.23   Developments in renal transplantation in the next 10 years will involve increases in living donor transplants, non-heart beating deceased donor transplants and combined pancreas-kidney transplants. There will also be an increase in transplantation for older patients with increased co-morbidity, and more emphasis on improvements in quality of life after transplantation. It is likely that there will be fewer transplant units in the UK, reflecting the need to optimise limited resources, in particular a shortage of transplant surgeons. In 2003, 21% of prevalent transplant patients were being followed up in RUs; this is likely to increase. The timing of transfer back to an RU from the RTU presently varies between 2 weeks and 12 months after transplantation, depending on clinical progress and local custom.

4.24   There is a need to identify renal physicians in RUs to give leadership for transplant medicine, recognising the increasing number of transplant patients being transferred for long-term follow-up from RTUs to RUs. The transplant physician's role would involve evaluation of potential live donors and transplant follow-up, as well as continuous professional development, training and research. Communication between RTUs and RUs that follow-up transplant patients must be maintained both by electronic and other communication, and also with visits to the RU from transplant surgeons and physicians based at the RTU.

4.25   There is a need to develop a subspecialty of transplant medicine. Additional experience in transplant medicine could be obtained after completion of renal medicine training and this should probably take at least one year. Such subspecialty training could benefit renal physicians appointed to consultant posts in RTUs, with an emphasis on acute transplantation, as well as those who will be lead transplant physicians in RUs.

RECOMMENDATION

We recommend the development of a subspecialty of transplant medicine.

Radiology

4.26   The need for support from radiology departments for imaging and interventional techniques including magnetic resonance and computerised tomographic angiography, renal angiography and angioplasty is increasing. Renal units vary in their need to access interventional radiology for insertion of dialysis catheters and renal biopsies. In some hospitals renal biopsies are performed by radiologists, so reducing opportunities for renal trainees to learn the technique.

Pathology

4.27   Specialist renal pathology expertise in reporting renal biopsies is essential to plan treatment for many types of renal disease. Clinico-pathological meetings of renal physicians and pathologists to discuss cases are a key part of clinical care, as well as an important CPD and training opportunity. This expertise may not be available on-site in all RUs, but should be provided by links with RTUs which ensure rapid transport of specimens, reporting of specimens within 24 hours for urgent cases, and regular clinico-pathological meetings either face to face or facilitated by videoconferencing.

Information technology

4.28   Renal clinical IT systems are essential for improving efficiency of clinical monitoring across managed clinical networks, clinical governance and audit, and returning accurate data to the Renal Association UK Renal Registry. Returns of data to the UK Renal Registry are mandated in England by the NSF. Not all renal units have either the infrastructure or appropriately trained informatics staff to support renal systems. Reliance on consultant renal physicians to provide routine systems management and analyses is inappropriate but funding to develop or upgrade

arrangements do not require the development of new roles such as consultant 'community nephrologists' or GPs with a special interest in renal medicine, but with education and mentoring, the wider primary care team can be educated and empowered to develop suitable care pathways for these patients.

4.49   Satellite haemodialysis facilities could be set up as part of or adjacent to primary care clinics, with general practitioners with a specialist interest in dialysis taking responsibility on a day-to-day basis for dialysis patients, on a shared care basis with hospital renal physicians. Periodic review of haemodialysis patients by general practitioners could occur within the satellite clinic setting, according to agreed care pathways.

RECOMMENDATION

We recommend joint working between the renal multiprofessional team, primary care and relevant specialist secondary care services promoting integrated care for patients with CKD, diabetes, vascular disease and for elderly patients and those patients who require conservative or palliative care. Consultant renal physicians should play a key leadership role in these service developments. These services should be in line with available clinical practice guidelines, and should be fully funded.

5 Commissioning of renal services

5.1   Renal services are 'specialised' services and are commissioned outside primary care trusts. The planning base for these services is a population of more than 1 million and is usually between 2 and 3 million. Commissioning includes assessing the population's health needs and securing services to meet these. This involves seeking views from all stakeholders; promoting diversity; balancing choice with clinical continuity; monitoring services against national standards; working with primary care colleagues and developing long-term strategic plans supported with investment.[31] Arrangements for commissioning of renal services for children are complex and distinct from the needs of adults.

5.2   Commissioners seek patient-led, patient-centred services with clear strategic direction and holistic care spanning patient pathways. They recognise that patients wish to use services located close to their homes with shared access to specialist centres where necessary, and the need to address problem areas, such as transport and vascular access surgery. Commissioners recognise the need for consultants to support general practitioners in developing pathways for identification and management of patients with CKD.

5.3   The current process for commissioning is variable across the country and in some areas there are significant service inequities which need to be addressed. Discussions led by specialised commissioners in some areas involve the full allocation of resources, while in others lead to a recommendation to primary care trusts to allocate resources. Published last year, the *Review of commissioning arrangements for specialised services* provides a framework for robust arrangements which if implemented could significantly improve commissioning of renal services.[32]

It is also recognised that the management of CKD is a broader commissioning issue which must be addressed across the patient pathway and responsible commissioning bodies.

5.4   Payment by Results requires the development of a national tariff; it is not anticipated that this will be in place for renal services until 2008.[33] Thus far the emphasis has been on developing tariffs for dialysis and transplantation, although there is as yet no consensus about which elements of care should be included. No tariffs have been proposed for other elements of renal care such as pre-dialysis care and non-dialysis care of advanced renal failure. In the future, developments will be funded from an allocation derived from the number of patients and the agreed tariff. However, the national tariff may not always reflect the local cost of services. The risk remains that funding received for renal services might continue to be allocated inappropriately elsewhere in a trust to meet deficits in other services.

5.5   If independent sector treatment centres (ISTCs) are developed for the provision of dialysis services, they should operate according to Royal College of Physicians/Renal Association standards within a clinical governance and quality assurance framework, allowing integrated and seamless transition of care between the ISTC and the NHS-funded renal service. In ISTC renal units, fully trained and accredited NHS renal physicians will provide the clinical lead to manage patients according to Royal College of Physicians/Renal Association standards. It is mandatory that maintenance of similar standards of care across public and private providers is rigorously audited.

RECOMMENDATIONS

We recommend an increased emphasis on the need for effective commissioning of renal services through locality networks, supported by a robust assessment of need and a prioritised investment plan.

We recommend that prevailing inequalities of provision of renal services are addressed, ensuring that the impact of ethnicity and social deprivation are properly identified when calculating funding.

We recommend that the tariff for renal services should be developed to properly reflect the cost of the complex activities of chronic disease management in renal care. This will require in depth clinical engagement.

We recommend that reference costs for pre-dialysis care and non-dialysis care of advanced renal failure are developed.

We recommend that all providers of renal services (including the NHS and the independent sector) should conform to RCP/Renal Association standards of care. It is crucial that maintenance of standards of care across public and private providers is rigorously audited.

Appendix

Witnesses

The Working Party is very grateful to the following people who gave their time to share experiences and offer advice, and to review an early draft of the report:

Lindsey Barker
Society for DGH Nephrologists

Rudy Bilous
Diabetes UK

Steve Blades
Royal College of General Practitioners

Susan Carr
SpR Programme Director, University Hospitals of Leicester NHS Trust

Fiona Dallas
Consultant Nephrologist, North Cumbria Hospitals NHS Trust

Bob Dunn
Advocacy Officer, National Kidney Federation

Chris Dudley
British Transplantation Society

Alison Ewing
Clinical Director of Pharmacy, Royal Liverpool and Broadgreen University Hospital Trust

Morag Gorrie
Renal Medicine Staff Grade and Associate Specialists Forum

Brian Junor
Scottish Renal Association

Fiona Karet
Professor of Renal Medicine, Cambridge Institute for Medical Research and University of Cambridge

Roop Kishen
Intensive Care Society

Jane MacDonald
British Renal Society

Heather Maxwell
British Association for Paediatric Nephrology

Peter Maxwell
Professor of Renal Medicine/Consultant Nephrologist, Belfast City Hospital

Fliss Murtagh
Association for Palliative Medicine

Shelagh O'Riordan
British Geriatric Society

Steven Powis
Chair, Specialty Advisory Committee for Renal Medicine

Charles Pusey
Kidney Research UK

Stuart Rodger
Clinical Director, Western Infirmary Glasgow

Paul Rylance
Society for DGH Nephrologists

Jenny Scott
Cheshire and Merseyside Specialist Services Commissioning Team

References

1 UK Renal Registry. *The Eighth Annual Report.* Bristol: UK Renal Registry. December 2005.

2 Federation of the Royal College of Physicians of the UK. *Census of consultant physicians in the UK, 2005: Data and commentary.* London: RCP, 2006.

3 Federation of the Royal Colleges of Physicians of the UK. *Census of consultant physicians in the UK, 2004: Data and commentary.* London: RCP, 2005.

4 The Renal Team. *A multiprofessional renal workforce plan for adults and children with renal disease: recommendations of the National Workforce Planning Group, 2002.* www.britishrenal.org

5 Royal Colleges of Physicians. *Consultant physicians working for patients: the duties, responsibilities and practice of physicians in general medicine and the specialties,* 3rd edn. London: RCP, 2004.

6 Postgraduate Medical Education and Training Board Regulations. *The General and Specialist Medical Practice* (Education, Training and Qualifications Order 2003 ISBN 0110460049 Statutory Instrument 2003 No 1,250)

7 Royal College of Physicians. *Training tomorrow's physicians: proposals from the Royal Colleges of Physicians on the training of specialists.* London: RCP, December 2005.

8 RCP specialist registrar career choices. www.rcplondon.ac.uk/professional/spr/spr_careerchoices.htm

9 The Academy of Medical Sciences. *The tenure-track clinician scientist: a new career pathway to promote recruitment into clinical academic medicine (Savill Report).* March 2000.
   www.academicmedicine.ac.uk/uploads/The%20tenure%20track%20clinician%20scientist.pdf

10 The Academy of Medical Sciences. *Clinical academic medicine in jeopardy: recommendations for change.* June 2002. www.academicmedicine.ac.uk/uploads/Academic%20Medicine%20in%20Jeopardy.pdf

11 The Academy of Medical Sciences. *Strengthening clinical research.* October 2003.
   www.academicmedicine.ac.uk/uploads/Strengthening%20Clinical%20Research.pdf

12 Royal College of Physicians. *Clinical academic medicine: the way forward.* A report from the forum on academic medicine. London: RCP, November 2004.
   www.academicmedicine.ac.uk/uploads/ClinAcadMed%20the%20way%20forward.pdf

13 Millbank Memorial Fund. *The future of academic medicine: five scenarios to 2025.* July 2005.
   www.academicmedicine.ac.uk/uploads/Milbank%20Fund%20report.pdf

14 The Council of Heads of Medical Schools. *Clinical academic staffing levels in UK medical and dental schools.* June 2005.
   www.chms.ac.uk/downloads/CHMS&CHDDS%20Survey%20of%20Clinical%20Academic%20Numbers%20June%202005.pdf

15 The Academy of Medical Sciences. *Medically- and dentally-qualified academic staff: Recommendations for training the researchers and educators of the future (Walport Report).* March 2005.
   www.mmc.nhs.uk/download/Medically-and-Dentally-Qualified-academic-staff-recommendations-Report.pdf

16 Department of Health. *Best research for best health: a new national health research strategy.* January 2006.
   www.dh.gov.uk/PublicationsAndStatistics/Publications/PublicationsPolicyAndGuidance/PublicationsPolicyAndGuidanceArticle/fs/en?CONTENT_ID=4127127&chk=uSh6qN

17   Department of Health. *The National Service Framework for Renal Services: part one: dialysis and transplantation.* London: Department of Health, January 2004.

18   Department of Health. *The National Service Framework for Renal Services: part two: chronic kidney disease, acute renal failure and end of life care.* London: Department of Health, February 2005.

19   The Renal Association. *Renal workforce recommendations: provision of services for adult patients with renal disease in the United Kingdom.* Bristol: The Renal Association.

20   National Institute of Health and Clinical Excellence. *Home haemodialysis: guidance on home compared with hospital haemodialysis for patients with end-stage renal failure.* October 2002.
www.nice.org.uk/page.aspx?o=TA048guidance

21   Rayner H, Greenwood R, Pisoni RL and Port FK. Haemodialysis in the UK – lessons learned from DOPPS. *Br J Renal Med* 2003;6–8.

22   Department of Health. *Modernising services for renal patients. Redesigning the workforce and re-engineering elective dialysis access surgery.* London: Department of Health, 2005.

23   Renal Workforce Competency Framework. **www.skillsforhealth.org.uk/frameworks.php**

24   National Institute for Health and Clinical Excellence. *Nutritional support in adults.* London: NICE, 2006.

25   British Association for Paediatric Nephrology. *Review of multiprofessional paediatric nephrology services in the UK – towards standards and equity of care: report of a working party of the British Association for Paediatric Nephrology,* 2003.

26   Department of Health. *Transition: getting it right for young people. Improving the transition of young people with long term conditions from children's to adult health services.* March 2006.
www.dh.gov.uk/PublicationsAndStatistics/Publications/PublicationsPolicyAndGuidance/Publications PolicyAndGuidanceArticle/fs/en?CONTENT_ID=4132145&chk=09SMKE

27   Department of Health. *National Service Framework for Diabetes.* London: Department of Health, 2001.

28   Royal College of Physicians. *Chronic kidney disease in adults: UK guidelines for identification, management and referral.* London: RCP, 2006.

29   Liverpool Care of the Dying Pathway (**www.lcp-mariecurie.org.uk/about**) Ellershaw J and Ward C. Care of the dying patient: the last hours or days of life. *BMJ,* 2003:326; 30–34.

30   Keri Thomas and Department of Health. Gold Standards Framework England 2005: NHS End of Life Care Programme. **www.goldstandardsframework.nhs.uk/index.php**

31   Department of Health. *Toolkit for commissioners of renal services.*
www.dh.gov.uk/PublicationsAndStatistics/Publications/PublicationsPolicyAndGuidance/Publications PolicyAndGuidanceArticle/fs/en?CONTENT_ID=4097227&chk=xa5YeD

32   Department of Health. *Review of commissioning arrangements for specialised services: an independent review.* May 2006.
www.dh.gov.uk/PolicyAndGuidance/HealthAndSocialCareTopics/SpecialisedServicesDefinition/ SpecialisedServicesDefinitionArticle/fs/en?CONTENT_ID=4001677&chk=/JlPYl

33   Department of Health. *Payment by Results.*
www.dh.gov.uk/PolicyAndGuidance/OrganisationPolicy/FinanceAndPlanning/NHSFinancialReforms/ fs/en